The 50/50 Diet

Count Calories. Exercise. Lose Weight.

by

MARTIN HARRIS

The 50/50 Diet

ISBN-13: 978-1517219703
ISBN-10: 1517219701

Dedication

Thanks to my wife for her support in writing this book and encouraging me to remain disciplined when I find it hard losing weight.

Thanks to J Sainsbury plc for giving permission to reproduce the nutritional information from their website.

Martin Harris
web: www.thefiftyfiftydiet.com
twitter: @fiftyfiftydiet
email: martin@thefiftyfiftydiet.com

Contents

Introduction

Losing weight and sticking to a diet is not easy. It takes discipline and patience. I'm full of enthusiasm and good intentions when I start a new diet but my bad habits soon return and my discipline evaporates. I tried 'Atkins' and it was great but then all I could think about was bread and rice and I soon stopped. I tried the '5:2 Diet'. That worked for a while, but eventually I forgot to do the '2' days. Lack of discipline again.

I've struggled with my weight since my teenage years. In 2012, I reached 23st (146kg). My energy levels were low, stamina was none existent and I got out of breath just climbing the stairs or walking to the train station. I love 'bad' food because it's convenient, cheap and tastes great.

I knew I had to change though - I didn't want to have a heart attack in my 40's. I'd tried various diets over the years with varying success. This time I kept it simple, I just ate fewer calories and started walking to get some exercise. Between 2012 and 2015, I lost about 4st (25kg).

So, you're probably thinking why aren't you writing about how you did that? Well, I never really had a plan. I just bumbled along, being good one month, bad the next. My weight loss wasn't controlled. I'm not sure I lost anything in 2013 or 2014. So, this time, I'm going to use what I learned and create a structured plan that gives me specific information and targets that I can follow and observe. This time, I want steady and continual weight loss.

Based on my experience of trying to lose weight, I came up with a few conclusions. Turning these conclusions into an actual plan that I could follow, led me to writing this book so other people could benefit. If this book helps just one other person lose weight, then it will have been a success.

The conclusions I came to were...
- I need to eat less.
- I need to eat better – stop eating junk food!
- I need to exercise more.
- I need to be patient.
- I need to maintain discipline.
- I mustn't give up.

When you look at it like this, what I'm actually talking about is a 'lifestyle change', not a diet. All I had to do was turn these conclusions into actions. So, that's what I did and I'll share it with you in this book.

Now, before we begin, a bit about me. I'm not a doctor, a nutritionist or a personal trainer. I'm not a reality star with an exercise DVD to promote. I'm not 10st (63kg) and I don't have a six-pack. Abercrombie & Fitch will never ask me to stand in front of their shops in my underpants. I'm not going to sell you some wonder treatment that will make the fat fall off your arse.

I'm quite ordinary. I'm a 45-year-old man that works as an IT Project Manager, organising computer projects for big companies, who just happens to have a lot of experience and disappointment with losing weight.

My greatest success came when I considered both food control and exercise. That's how I came up with the title for this book, 'The 50/50 Diet'. One of my conclusions was that counting calories will only get you 50% of the way. Dieting alone is too hard. You have to include exercise for the other 50% to burn more calories. I think many diets fail because they are too restrictive and they just focus on the food aspect. They only consider the calories 'in', not the calories 'out'.

I began to think, there must be a point where calories 'in' and calories 'out' meet in the middle. Where everything we eat is used up and our weight would remain the same. If I knew where that middle point was, I should be able to tweak the number of calories to create a shortfall, forcing my body to turn fat back into energy, therefore losing weight. Fortunately, some very clever scientists worked out how to find that 'middle' point and they were kind enough to write down a formula. In this book, I'll show you how to calculate the all-important numbers that will need to create your diet plan. Don't worry if you aren't good at maths. I'll give you a website you can go to that does the maths for you.

It's important to note that this diet is about focusing on how much you eat and not what you eat. It's different to other diets like Atkins, South Beach or Paleo for example. With my diet, you can eat anything you want. Nothing is off limits. You just have to control how much of you eat, which to be fair, will limit your enjoyment of really high calorie food. I can promise you though, that there are no gimmicks, no crazy ideas, no miracle cures and no expensive pre-prepared food to buy.

I have developed a plan that anyone can use, that is sensible, healthy with the objective to help you lose around 2lb (0.9kg) per week. That's half a stone (4kg) a month. You just need to do some simple maths, count the calories, stay within your calorie limit and exercise.

Chapter One
Lifestyle Change

So, we need to make some changes. Cut back on the bad food, eat healthier, do more exercise. Not only will these things help our waistlines but they will improve our overall health. We want long-term, sustainable weight loss, so I'm afraid it means saying goodbye to some of our favourite things that got us where we are today.

What's the Objective?

Easy! To lose weight, but we should do it in a way that is sensible, safe and healthy. Why? Well, we don't want to make ourselves ill and we want the weight to stay off. When you stop following a strict diet, it's typical for the weight to come back because all you did was amend your lifestyle for a short period. All you got for your effort is a short-term result. We want long-term results.

What Are the Timescales?

The 50/50 Diet plan will require you to make a long-term commitment. You probably spent years putting the weight on like I did. It will take time to lose it, so you need to be patient. With this plan, the aim is to lose around 2lb (0.9kg) per week. This is a safe and sustainable amount of weight to lose every week.

How Much Can You Lose?

How much is entirely up to you and there is no limit. This diet will work just as well if you want to lose 6st (40kg) or if you want to lose ½ st (3kg). Why? Because you are deliberately creating a shortfall in the calories your body needs, causing it to burn fat. This principle doesn't change whilst you follow your plan, regardless of how long you stay on the plan.

What Will You Have to Do?

Following The 50/50 Diet will require you to put some effort and planning into it.

You will have to count calories

- Buy some kitchen scales so you can measure food quantities. I use a digital one I bought on Amazon for £16.
- One of the biggest reason for gaining weight is we eat too much. The scales will help you measure and control food quantities.
- Use apps / websites like MyFitnessPal to record what you eat.

Start cooking more of your meals

- Preparing and cooking your own food, gives you complete control over the calories you consume.

- You don't need to be too adventurous. Look at the back of this book for recipe ideas, use Google to search for 'low calorie meals', buy a cookbook from your local book store.

- There are lots of low-calorie recipes available.

Your body can survive on far fewer calories

- You will learn how many calories your body really needs to function and I don't mean surviving at the point of starvation. No, I mean living a normal, busy life.

- It's probably a lot less than you eat now.

Drink more water

- Drink more water. Try to drink 2 litres a day.

- Being thirsty is often mistaken for hunger, leading us to eat when our bodies don't actually need food.

You will need to be disciplined

- You will get hungry sometimes.

- You will feel like a chocolate bar or cheeseburger.

- Try drinking water or a cup of tea then waiting 10 minutes. If you still feel hungry, then have a low calorie snack until your next meal.

You will need to be patient

- You built up this weight over time.
- It will take time to lose it in a healthy way.
- By employing a healthier lifestyle, you are much more likely to keep the weight off, because you've removed many of your bad habits.

You won't have to give up any food

- You can still keep your social life, drink beer and wine and go to restaurants. You just need to stay within your daily calorie limit.
- If you're going out, plan your day so you eat lightly and save your calories for later.
- In restaurants, sacrifice bad food you can do without, like chips or onion rings. Swap high calorie cake for a scoop of ice cream. You needn't let the diet ruin your night out.
- Remember too, that one bad day won't ruin your long-term plan.

You will learn new things about food

- Hopefully you'll be more educated about food.
- You will know which types of food and brands are good and which are bad. Which are high in sugar and salt, which should be your first choice food to buy and eat.

Chapter Two
All About Me

To make the next section where you calculate your diet plan easier to understand, I thought it would be useful if I give you a real-life example, so you can see how the calculations are done. So, I'm going to use my own personal body information as the example.

So this is me. I am 45 and I weigh 19st 11lb (126kg).

"Huh? Wait! What!? Almost 20st (127kg). You're not 12st (80kg) with a rippling six-pack, you haven't lost 50% of your bodyweight and you don't have a career as an underwear model? Why am I reading a book by you about losing weight?"

It's a fair question. Well, the answer is I know quite a lot about dieting as it happens and I've learned even more whilst I researched food and exercise for this book. Would you prefer to read about losing weight from a skinny gym-rat who has never been overweight in their life and a hard body that is simply depressing to the rest of us, or a loud-mouthed TV personality that thinks losing 3st (19kg) is easy and fat people are just lazy?

I'm the same as you. I understand the daily battle between desire and discipline. I have a lot of experience of what doesn't work and I've learned what does. At my biggest, I was 23st (146kg). I'm less now, so I know this 50/50 Diet Plan works and I'm still doing it until I hit my target weight.

What you get in this book is an honest approach to losing weight, by someone who is doing it right now and not just talking about it. I'm still overweight and I'm going to try my best to follow my own advice. You want to see proof if the 50/50 Diet works? Well you can.

You can follow me on Twitter **@FiftyFiftyDiet**, where I'll post comments about my progress, ideas and food suggestions. I personally respond to any messages that people send me.

You can also see what food I've been eating and how my weight loss is progressing, on MyFitnessPal's website. Search for my username **'martinharris10'** then follow me. I'll record everything I eat, honestly, even if I'm bad.

So, Day 1. It's 8am, Friday 1st January 2016 and I've just weighed myself…

- Weight, 19st 11lb (126.0kg)
- Height, 6 feet 0 inches tall (1.83m)
- Gender, Male
- Age, 45

It's a bigger number than I wanted to see if I'm honest, but there it is. It's the truth. If I follow my plan (which I will show you how to create in the next chapter), my weight will be less in just seven days.

BMI

According to the UK National Health Service website,

http://www.nhs.uk/Tools/Pages/Healthyweightcalculator.aspx

I am categorised as 'obese'. If there is ever a word in the English language that installs depression and actually has a demotivating effect, this is it. However, don't worry because BMI is a flawed measurement.

It groups the population into four categories, labelling us 'underweight', 'normal', 'overweight' or 'obese'. It takes no account of genetics or lifestyle. It's simply ratio of weight and height.

Bodybuilders and rugby players often get classified as obese because they have low levels of body fat but lots of dense muscle which weighs more than fat. Do they look like they need to lose weight? No.

So, up yours BMI.

What Should You Focus on Then?

There are many more useful things you can focus on to monitor progress, rather than your BMI number.

The most obvious and one you will do on a daily or weekly basis, is stand on the bathroom scales. Even when you've been good, the number can fluctuate, but over the long-term, we want to see it going down.

I find that clothes are a useful indicator too. How do your clothes fit you now? If you have a shirt that makes your stomach look like a caterpillar when you button it up don't throw it away. Put it at the back of your closet for three months then try it on again. Are you still the same caterpillar or does it feel looser and more comfortable?

Make a note which notch on your belt you use. You'll feel really happy when you have to go on eBay and buy a belt hole cutting gadget because the last remaining hole no longer holds your trousers up.

One of the most noticeable things I ever experienced was on an aeroplane flight. I hadn't been on one since I was at my biggest. Considering this was economy class, I was amazed that (a) I could comfortably sit in the chair, (b) I could fasten the seat belt without having to suck in every stomach muscle I possess, (c) when the stewardess walked down the aisle to check every passenger's seatbelt was fastened, she could see mine was done up because my stomach was no longer spilling over the seatbelt obscuring her view, and (d) I could fold the food tray down flat, because my stomach didn't get in the way, stopping it at a 45-degree angle.

All these things are visual markers you can use to monitor weight loss. For me wearing an item of clothing that now feels really comfortable is really satisfying.

The easiest method is of course weighing yourself. I tend to do it almost every day and record it on MyFitnessPal. I find it helps me retain discipline to be good. If I'm not good for one day and I see the number go up, it's like a kick up the arse to be good again. I have my 'big' weigh in, first thing every Friday morning. The key is to follow the same routine each time you weigh yourself, so that you are measuring a constant,

e.g. Friday morning because I tend to be better over the week than I am over the weekend, as soon as I get up, use the toilet first to lose a few extra ounces/grams and before the morning cup of tea and breakfast.

Chapter Three

Part One of the Plan: Calorie Control

In this chapter, I'll show you how to build the first part of the 50/50 Diet Plan. 'Calorie Control'.

You will…

- Calculate how many calories your body needs
- Choose your target weight
- Calculate the amount of weight you need to lose
- Calculate how long it will take to lose
- Calculate the maximum number of calories you can eat every day
- Plot your timeline plan

If you get stuck at any stage trying to calculate your Diet Plan, don't give up. Just email me I'll help you.

martin@martinharris10.com

Step 1 of 5
Calculate Your BMR

Let's begin. The medical profession recommends women eat 2,000 calories a day and men 2,500 calories. These are easy to remember numbers, but not the exact number your body actually needs. Everyone is different. Height, gender, age, medical condition and activity levels all affect how many calories our bodies need.

There are two ways to calculate how many calories your body needs:

1. The easy way – use someone's website.
2. The hard way – do the maths yourself.

I'll show you both.

The Easy Way

The number of calories your body needs just to function and keep you alive is known as the 'Basal Metabolic Rate'. There are lots of websites that let you input your stats and they calculate your BMR for you. I use MyFitnessPal's website. It's very easy to use.

http://www.myfitnesspal.com/tools/bmr-calculator

MyFitnessPal.com is a great website. It's free to use and is great for recording the food you eat and calculating how many calories you consume, but it also has other features, like calculating your BMR.

Input your details and click the 'Calculate' button. These are mine…

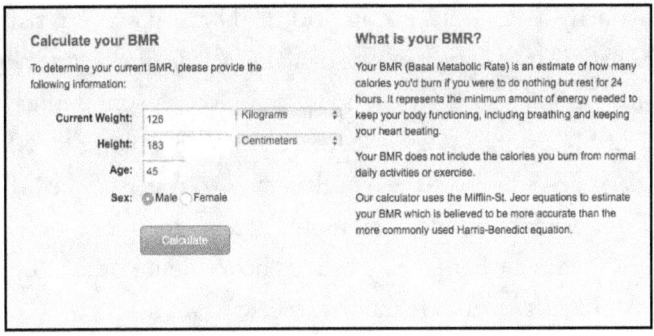

This is my result…

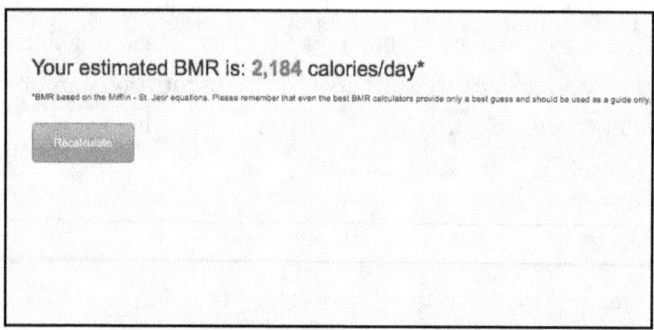

So, I should be eating **2,184** calories every day.

Record this number because you'll need it later.

The Government and medical professionals recommend as a man I should eat around 2,500 calories every day. That's 316 calories more than the calculation based on my personal stats says I should eat. Doesn't sound much, but 316 calories a day, soon becomes 9,480 calories in 30-days. So, you can see why calculating your personal BMR is so important and you should ignore the nice, round, Government numbers. Theirs is better than nothing, but BMR calculations are much more accurate.

The Hard Way

If you want to calculate your BMR value yourself, here's how. Just like the MyFitnessPal webpage I used, I will show you the equation produced by people smarter than myself. It's called the 'Mifflin – St. Jeor' equation.

1st - Convert Your Measurements into Metric

- To convert stones into pounds, multiply by 14.
- To convert pounds into kilos, divide by 2.2
- To convert feet into inches, multiply by 12.
- To convert inches into centimetres, multiply inches by 2.54

e.g. In Imperial measurements, I weigh 18st 12lb and I'm 6' 0" tall. This is how I convert them to metric numbers.

WEIGHT

- 19 stones x 14 = 266 pounds
- Add the remaining 11 pounds
- My total weight is 277 pounds
- 277 divided by 2.2, equals 125.9kg

HEIGHT

- 6 feet x 12 = 72 inches
- There are no remaining inches to add
- My total height is 72 inches.
- 72 x 2.54, equals 182.88. I'll round it up to 183cm

2nd - Apply the Formula

Apply your weight and height in metric, and your age, to the formula for men or women below.

Women
```
(10 x weight in kg) + (6.25 x height in cm) -
(5 x age in yrs) - 161
```

Men
```
(10 x weight in kg) + (6.25 x height in cm) -
(5 x age in yrs) + 5
```

Let's work out my BMR...

My weight is **19st 11lb** or **277lb.**

I'm 6' tall or **72"** and I'm **45.**

In metric measurements, that's **126kg** and **183cm.**

Using the equation for a man, my BMR is...
```
(10 x 126) + (6.25 x 183) - (5 x 45) + 5 =
2,183.75. Round it up to 2,184.
```

So, you can do the maths yourself or use someone else's website to do it for you. I use the MyFitnessPal website. The easy way.

Choose Your Target Weight

Next, if you have a target weight in mind, that's great. If you don't, you can use websites again to help you. I use the UK's NHS website…

http://www.nhs.uk/Tools/Pages/Healthyweightcalculator.aspx

You will need to choose 'adult' and your gender, then input your age, height and current weight. You can enter these numbers in metric or imperial.

Next, choose your typical level of daily activity. I work in an office every day and either get the train or drive to work, so I selected 'I am inactive'.

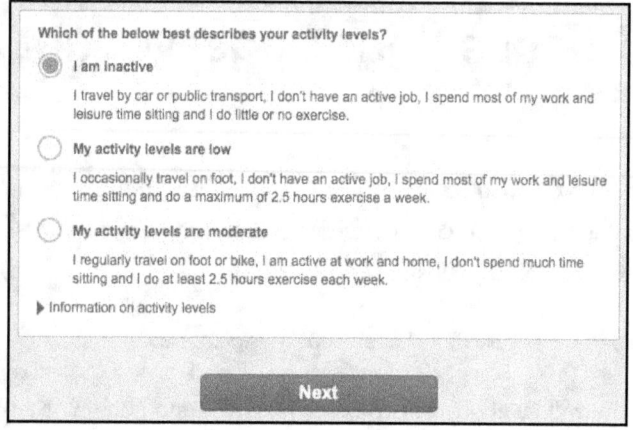

Which of the below best describes your activity levels?

○ **I am inactive**

I travel by car or public transport, I don't have an active job, I spend most of my work and leisure time sitting and I do little or no exercise.

○ **My activity levels are low**

I occasionally travel on foot, I don't have an active job, I spend most of my work and leisure time sitting and do a maximum of 2.5 hours exercise a week.

○ **My activity levels are moderate**

I regularly travel on foot or bike, I am active at work and home, I don't spend much time sitting and I do at least 2.5 hours exercise each week.

▶ Information on activity levels

Next

The website then calculates your ideal weight range.

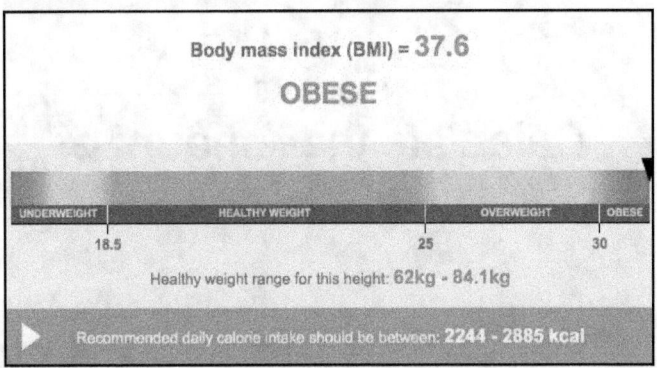

Ignore the BMI score and the rude message that says I'm 'obese'.

I'm interested in the bit below that, where it says 'healthy weight range for this height is 9st 11lb – 13st 3lb (62kg to 84.1kg)'. I'm going to choose **12st 7lb (80kg)** as my target weight. It's an easy number to remember and puts me in the 'healthy weight' range.

Use the website to see what it recommends your ideal weight range is and choose a number you are happy with. If you don't like what the website tells you, ignore it. Choose your own target weight. It's your plan.

Calculate the Amount of Weight to Lose

I want to be 12st 7lb (80kg) and you know what weight you want to be. The next step is a simple calculation to work out how much you need to lose, to get from where you are now to where you want to be.

I'm 19st 11lb (126kg), so my calculation is...

```
19st 11lb - 12st 7lb = 7st 4lb
126kg - 80kg = 46kg
```

Losing 7st 4lb (46kg) sounds impossible, but that's OK. That's my target weight loss over the duration of the plan. I'm not aiming to lose it all in a month.

Do the same maths with your current weight minus your target weight, to calculate the total amount of weight you want to lose.

Step 4 of 5

Calculate How Long It Will Take

Now this is the part most people want to focus on – how long will it take to lose the weight?

This diet is NOT a miracle cure. It's a balance of weight loss through cutting back a sensible amount of calories every day and increasing exercise levels to burn more calories, combined to maximise your weight loss, but in a controlled, sustainable and safe way.

So, we know how much weight we want to lose. I want to lose 7st 4lb (46kg). How much is a sensible and safe amount to lose each week?

Medical professionals would advise no more than 2lb (0.9kg) per week, so this is what we are going to aim for.

The, it's back to the maths…

- I want to lose 7st 4lb (46kg) in total.
- I want to lose 2lb (0.9kg) per week.
- Divide 'weight to lose' by 2lb (0.9kg).
- It will take me 51 weeks to lose 102lb (46kg).

If I can achieve that, it would be really good but it will require me to be disciplined for 12 months. I know I'm not going to be perfect, so it might take a bit longer, but I'll do my best to hit my target on New Year's Eve 2016.

Now, you do the maths for your stats.

- You know how much you want to lose.
- Aim to lose 2lb (0.9kg) a week
- Divide the amount you want to lose by 2lb (0.9kg) to tell you how many weeks it will take.
- Add a bit more time on because you'll have bad days too.

Step 5 of 5

Calculate the Maximum Number of Daily Calories

Step 5, the final step. You know how much you want to lose and how long it will take. Now we work out how you are going to achieve this weight loss. Up until now, it's about what you want to do. This is where we work out the how.

We are aiming to lose 2lb (0.9kg) per week. This is our total weekly weight loss, but we're not going to lose it through dieting alone. It needs to be split 50/50 between calorie control and exercise.

So for the calorie calculations, we want to lose 1lb (0.5kg) per week.

OK, so how many calories are there in 1lb (0.5kg) of fat? The answer is about 3,500 calories, which works out very nicely to 500 a day.

If you want to see the maths, clever people have worked it out for us.

- 1lb is 454 grams
- Fat has 9 calories per gram
- Human fat tissue is about 87% actual fat.
- Therefore, 454g (1lb) of body fat tissue is 395g of pure fat (454g x 87%).
- Multiply 395g by 9 calories per gram and you get 3,555 calories.
- Round it to 3,500 to make the maths simpler.

We want to lose 1lb (0.5kg) of weight, every week, through cutting back on food intake. So, we need to knock 500 calories off our daily calorie allowance (3,500 calories divided by 7 days)

Look at the BMR (Basal Metabolic Rate) figure you calculated for yourself in step one. Mine was **2,184** calories. This is my daily calorie amount to maintain my present weight, but I want to lose 1lb (0.5kg) every week by reducing calorie intake, so I need to subtract the 500 calories we just worked out. My daily calorie limit must not exceed **1,684 calories** (2,184 – 500).

Work out what your maximum daily calorie limit is by subtracting 500 calories from your BMR.

You can set your maximum calorie intake on your MyFitnessPal profile, by…

Going to http://www.myfitnesspal.com

- Log on or create an account.
- In the menus going across the top of the screen, 'My Home' should already be highlighted.
- Click 'Goals' beneath it.
- The webpage will change to display three tables; daily goals, fitness and micronutrients.
- In the 'Daily Goals' section, click the 'Edit' button.
- Type in the maximum number of daily calories you calculated. Mine was 1,684.
- Set Carbohydrates to 40%
- Set Fat to 30%
- Set Protein to 30%
    - o Aim for this balance in the food you eat and it will give you a well-balanced diet.
    - o You'll probably need to eat fewer carbs and eat more veg and protein.
    - o Don't worry about fat being 30%. Some fats are good for you. They're not all bad.
- Click the 'Save Changes' button.

Summary

OK, so you've gone through all the steps of the plan and you should have all your information. This was mine.

- Target weight: **12st 7lb** (80kg)
- Amount to lose: **7st 4lb or 102lb** (46kg)
- Duration: **51 weeks**
- Maximum no. daily calories: **1,684**

Plot your target weight-loss weekly, so you know where you aim to be each week. I do my 'big, end of week' weigh-in, every Friday morning. The table on the next page shows where I aim to be at the end of each month. I know some months are longer than others, but it's only a rough guide.

Tip: Print this out and stick it up somewhere visible, so it's a constant reminder.

This is my monthly target:

Now: 1st January 2016	19st 11lb	126kg
31 January 2016	18st 8lb	122kg
29 February 2016	18st 4lb	118kg
31 March 2016	17st 9lb	114kg
30 April 2016	17st 0lb	110kg
31 May 2016	16st 5lb	106kg
30 June 2016	15st 10lb	102kg
31 July 2016	15st 2lb	98kg
31 August 2016	14st 7lb	94kg
30 September 2016	13st 12lb	90kg
31 October 2016	13st 3lb	86kg
30 November 2016	12st 8lb	82kg
31 December 2016	13st 3lb	80kg

Do your best to stick to this new calorie limit every day and you should achieve 50% of your weight loss goal.

If I can stick to 1,684 calories every day, this should equate to roughly 3st 8lb (23kg) of weight loss – just by knocking off 500 calories a day.

Chapter Four

Part Two of the Plan: Exercise

In the last chapter we calculated the daily food intake to earn 50% of our weight loss goal. Now, in Part Two, exercise will earn us the other 50%.

This chapter will look at different types of exercise you can do at home, so you don't have to join an expensive gym. I'm going categorise exercises into two groups and call them 'Non-Gym' and 'Home Gym'. 'Non-gym' exercise is carrying out activity that you wouldn't normally associate as exercise, like gardening, cleaning or playing sports. 'Home-Gym' is exercises that you can easily transfer from a gym and do in the privacy of your own home, without the expense of gym membership.

Sleep

Before I talk about exercise, I want to cover sleep.

Medical experts now agree than sleep plays a very important function in human health and weight control. Whilst you are asleep your body is still working hard. Your body releases hormones that help repair cells and control the body's use of energy. These hormonal changes can affect your body weight. Sleep affects growth and stress hormones, the immune system, appetite, breathing, blood pressure and cardiovascular health. Cutting out a couple of hours of sleep on a regular basis can have a significant impact on your health. Lack of sleep reduces your ability to solve problems, reasoning and attention to detail, it impacts your mood and how you interact with others.

So, how much sleep is the right amount? On average, adults ought to get 7 to 8 hours of sleep every night. However, sleep can easily be disrupted, so try to avoid stimulants like caffeine before going to bed and it's now thought that the light emitted from electronic devices can affect the quality of your sleep, so try limiting the use of phones, tablets and TVs in the bedroom.

Safety Warning About Exercise

If you have any medical conditions, consult your doctor before taking up exercise. Remember to be safe and sensible when you exercise. Don't go for the heaviest weights or aim to run long distances immediately. You'll hurt yourself. Find the level of exercise that feels comfortable and then slowly build up over time, to burn more calories, to encourage greater weight loss.

You probably spent a long time gaining the weight you have. It won't come off immediately. Remember my plan? To lose weight over a year? Our exercise goal is to burn 500 calories a day, not become a bodybuilder who can bench-press the weight of a small car or represent our country at the next Olympics.

Look at the exercises listed over the next few pages, see how many calories they burn and choose one or two that suit your lifestyle and ability.

Exercise safely. If it hurts, stop!

Non-Gym Exercise

There are plenty of exercises you can do without using a gym. Walking the dog, hiking, golf, tennis, swimming, washing the car, gardening, it's all exercise. Here are the average numbers of calories you burn in 30 minutes.

Figures were obtained from MyFitnessPal.com

Walking/Jogging
Walking (leisurely – 15mins/km), 177 kcals
Walking (brisk – 10mins/km), 224 kcals
Jogging (gentle - 10.7 kph, 5.6min/km), 649 kcals
Jogging (brisk – 14.5 kph, 4.1min/km, 885 kcals

Household
Cleaning (light, moderate effort), 148 kcals
Cleaning (heavy, vigorous effort), 177 kcals
Gardening, general, 236 kcals

Sports
Golf (carrying clubs), 266 kcals
Tennis (doubles), 295 kcals
Swimming (freestyle, moderate effort), 413 kcals
Cycling (moderate – 19-23 kph), 472 kcals
Football (competitive), 531 kcals
Swimming (breaststroke), 590 kcals
Rugby, 590 kcals

You can see it's easy to get 500 calories worth of exercise.

- 1 hour of brisk walking
- 30 mins of jogging
- 1 hour of gardening
- 30 mins of cycling at a moderate pace
- 30 mins of swimming

The easiest is walking or jogging. I walk. According to RunKeeper, walking at a brisk pace for **5km (3.1 miles) = 500 calories**. If you don't have time to walk this far in one session, break it up into smaller walks. Alternatively, install a pedometer app on your smart phone and aim to walk at least **8,000 steps every day**. That will get you to the 500 calories. How do you define a 'brisk' walk? Elevated heart rate, slight sweating but still being able to talk as you walk.

There are apps you can use to record your walks, that monitor the time, distance and estimate the number of calories you burn. I use RunKeeper. It links to MyFitnessPal, so it feeds the exercise you do into your diet plan. There are lots of other apps out there too, for both iPhone and Android.

Find an exercise that you enjoy that fits your daily routine.

Home-Gym Exercise

There are many exercises that you can take from the gym and safely do at home, with little or no equipment. This is more than just doing the housework or gardening. It is gym-style exercise, without the need for an expensive membership.

I will describe a series of exercises that work the legs, the stomach and arms, to give an all-over body workout, set over a month. As I've said before, I'm not a fitness expert. I found these exercises on the Internet when I was researching exercise that I could do at home. They are easy to find. Use Google to search for "30-day exercise plan". I try to follow the plan I will show you combined with walking, to boost the calories I burn.

The plan starts small, listing exercises to do every 4 days, then you have a rest day. The difficulty factor builds up each day, increasing the number of times you repeat the exercises. If you reach a point where you find the exercise level is hard going, it's OK to stay at that level. Find the level you feel comfortable with and only progress to the next level when you feel capable. Train safely. If you stay at a given level for a few days (or longer), don't forget to take every 4th day as a rest day where you do no exercise.

The exercises I'll describe are designed to work on strengthening and conditioning your muscles because bigger, healthy muscles need more bloody supply, more oxygen and burn more calories. Ladies, you won't end up like a bodybuilder, so don't worry. Those girls and guys train for years to look like that. These exercises will help you lose weight and improve the tone and shape of your muscles. You won't turn into Miss Universe. That takes years of dedication and hours and hours in the gym.

The only money I spent to do these exercises, was buying two 10kg dumbbells on Amazon, for about £40.

One more tip. Chaps, if you are looking for exercises that will give you a six-pack – it doesn't exist. You already have a six-pack. They're your stomach muscles. You just can't see them because of the layer of fat covering them. The only way to reveal your six-pack is to burn calories and reduce the amount of body fat you have so they become visible. Ignore promises of magic results with minimal effort. They dangle the dream but never deliver.

My 30-day Home Gym Routine

This is the additional exercise routine I try to do as well as walking. The walking gives me my 500 calorie target but this burns bonus calories increasing weight loss and will also improve muscle definition and make me look sexy. Well, that's the idea. Ask the wife in one year if she thinks I'm sexy. Probably not.

There are lots of exercise plans available on the Internet for free. I searched Google Images for "30-day challenge" and found these. The plans are clearly laid out, they show the amount of exercise to attempt and there are pictures to show you how to perform each exercise.

30-day Chest Challenge:
https://www.pinterest.com/pin/150941024986530188/

30-day Butt Challenge:
https://www.pinterest.com/pin/150941024986530184/

30-day Shoulder Challenge:
https://www.pinterest.com/pin/150941024984912689/

30-day Thigh Challenge:
https://www.pinterest.com/pin/150941024984740983/

30-Day Back Challenge:
https://www.pinterest.com/pin/150941024984441139/

30-Day Arm Challenge:
https://www.pinterest.com/pin/150941024983921913/

I don't have time to do every single challenge, as well as go to work every day and do walking. Also, I don't need to do every 30-day Challenge (no-one is saying I have to). I want to work my stomach area and upper body. I'm perfectly happy with my legs and arse.

So, I mixed and matched different pieces from different 30-day challenges to make my own custom-made one. You can do the same too. Focus on the parts of your body you want to improve and chose a maximum of 8-10 different exercises you can do at home.

You can see pictures of the exercises on the links I just gave you or search YouTube.com to watch videos.

A few tips…

Tip 1: When the numbers get bigger, don't try to do all of them in one go. The professionals break the overall target into sets and repetitions. They will do the exercise a small number of times (called 'sets') and repeat it ('reps') until they hit the total number they want to achieve.

e.g. on Day10, I am supposed to do 50 sit-ups. Doing this all in one go will hurt the next day, so I do 10 sit-ups then rest and repeat this 5 times, to get to the 50.

Tip 2: Exercise safely. If you reach a level that you feel is your limit and you cannot do anymore, then don't. Stay at that level every day (except rest days), until and feel you can try for the next level. It's not a competition. You're not training for the Olympics. Listen to your body and if it hurts, then stop. Exercise safely.

This is my custom 30-day challenge, where I focus on arms, stomach and shoulders. I mix the exercises up so I work one set of muscles as another set takes a rest.

		Day 1	2	3	4
Leg raises	Abs	5	8	10	
Push ups	Arms	5	8	10	R
Crunches	Abs	5	8	10	E
Dips	Arms	5	8	10	S
Shoulder Press	Shoulders	10	15	20	T
Bicep curls	Arms	10	15	20	
Sit ups	Abs	15	20	25	D
Plank	Abs	10s	12s	15s	A
Upright row	Shoulders	10	15	25	Y
Side lateral raise	Shoulders	5	8	10	

		Day 5	6	7	8
Leg raises	Abs	12	15	20	
Push ups	Arms	12	15	18	R
Crunches	Abs	12	15	20	E
Dips	Arms	15	20	25	S
Shoulder Press	Shoulders	30	40	50	T
Bicep curls	Arms	30	40	50	
Sit ups	Abs	30	35	40	D
Plank	Abs	20s	25s	30s	A
Upright row	Shoulders	35	45	50	Y
Side lateral raise	Shoulders	15	20	25	

		Day 9	10	11	12
Leg raises	Abs	30	30	33	
Push ups	Arms	20	22	25	R
Crunches	Abs	30	50	65	E
Dips	Arms	30	35	40	S
Shoulder Press	Shoulders	55	60	65	T
Bicep curls	Arms	55	60	65	
Sit ups	Abs	45	50	55	D
Plank	Abs	35s	38s	42s	A
Upright row	Shoulders	60	70	75	Y
Side lateral raise	Shoulders	30	35	40	

		Day 13	14	15	16
Leg raises	Abs	40	42	42	
Push ups	Arms	28	29	30	R
Crunches	Abs	75	85	90	E
Dips	Arms	50	55	60	S
Shoulder Press	Shoulders	75	80	85	T
Bicep curls	Arms	75	80	85	
Sit ups	Abs	60	65	70	D
Plank	Abs	50s	55s	60s	A
Upright row	Shoulders	80	90	95	Y
Side lateral raise	Shoulders	50	55	60	

		Day 17	18	19	20
Leg raises	Abs	45	48	50	
Push ups	Arms	35	36	38	R
Crunches	Abs	100	110	120	E
Dips	Arms	65	70	75	S
Shoulder Press	Shoulders	90	100	105	T
Bicep curls	Arms	90	100	105	
Sit ups	Abs	75	80	85	D
Plank	Abs	65s	70s	75s	A
Upright row	Shoulders	100	105	110	Y
Side lateral raise	Shoulders				

		Day 21	22	23	24
Leg raises	Abs	52	55	58	
Push ups	Arms	40	42	44	R
Crunches	Abs	130	140	150	E
Dips	Arms	80	85	90	S
Shoulder Press	Shoulders	110	115	120	T
Bicep curls	Arms	110	115	120	
Sit ups	Abs	90	95	100	D
Plank	Abs	80s	85s	90s	A
Upright row	Shoulders	120	125	130	Y
Side lateral raise	Shoulders				

		Day 25	26	27	28
Leg raises	Abs	60	60	62	
Push ups	Arms	45	46	47	R
Crunches	Abs	160	170	180	E
Dips	Arms	95	100	105	S
Shoulder Press	Shoulders	125	130	135	T
Bicep curls	Arms	125	130	135	
Sit ups	Abs	105	110	115	D
Plank	Abs	95s	100s	110s	A
Upright row	Shoulders	140	145	150	Y
Side lateral raise	Shoulders	95	100	105	

		Day 29	30		
Leg raises	Abs	62	65		
Push ups	Arms	48	50		
Crunches	Abs	190	200		
Dips	Arms	110	120		
Shoulder Press	Shoulders	140	150		
Bicep curls	Arms	140	150		
Sit ups	Abs	120	125		
Plank	Abs	115s	120s		
Upright row	Shoulders	160	175		
Side lateral raise	Shoulders	110	120		

The 50/50 Diet Summarised

Now you've seen how to calculate your 50/50 Diet plan.

- Aim to lose 2lb (0.9kg) a week or 7,000 calories
- Split this weight loss goal 50/50 between calorie control and exercise
- Cut your food intake back by 500 calories a day
- Exercise every day to burn another 500 calories

CALORIE CONTROL:
- Calculate how many calories your body needs
- Choose your target weight
- Calculate the amount of weight you need to lose
- Calculate how long it will take you to lose
- Calculate the maximum number of calories you can eat every day
- Plot your timeline plan

EXERCISE:
- Choose exercises that you enjoy

Chapter Five
Food

This chapter is going to take you through a study I have done about food. It's not a deeply scientific study, so don't worry.

Hopefully, it will improve your understanding about food chemistry, you'll learn how to read and understand food labels and then there are pages of similar food types sorted by their calorie value, to make it easier for you to see which products have lower and higher calorie values. This will help you choose what you eat and stay inside your daily calorie limit.

Current Thinking

There is so much confusion about food these days. For the last thirty years, the message has been to eat a low fat diet, but now the current enemy is not fat, it is sugar. Sugar added to processed food.

We're making a calorie controlled diet, where we can eat anything we want but we have to stick within our daily calorie limit. By being selective about the food we choose to eat, we can maximise the quantity we can eat, helping us feel fuller for longer and improve our health by avoiding the foods that aren't very good for us, like heavily processed foods which are often high in bad fats, sugar and calories.

I advocate eating as much meat, fruit and vegetables and as little processed food as possible. Food manufacturers add all kinds of chemicals to processed food to make it taste better, make it last longer and make it look more attractive, but it's not as good for us as more natural food. Cooking your own food, using as few processed ingredients as possible, gives you greater control of the calories and quality of the food you eat.

Macro & Micronutrients

Let's start with a little chemistry about food. Food is made up of macro and micronutrients. Macronutrients are the big stuff that provides your body with energy (calories), carbohydrate, fat and protein. Alcohol provides calories but it's not considered to be a macronutrient as it is not required for health. Micronutrients are the small stuff, like vitamins and minerals. It's important to eat carbs, protein and fat in the right proportions, so that you have a balanced diet. Too much of one type can lead to health problems. Government guidelines recommend adults consume approximately...

- 40% of calories from carbohydrates
- 30% from fat
- 30% from protein

This balance is fine for most people but some groups, like children and pregnant women, will need to adjust these levels.

If you use an app like MyFitnessPal, you can set your daily calorie intake level and the ratio of carbs, protein and fat you want to eat. As you record the food you eat, it will show you how many calories and how much of each nutrient you still have left to eat. After a while, you will begin using apps like these, to check the values of food, before you consume them, to help you stay within your limits. It becomes habitual.

Carbohydrates

There's a misconception that carbohydrates make you fat. It's not true. As we've learned, if you eat more calories than your body needs, you gain weight, not because of which food type you eat. Carbs are a healthy part of your diet and should be included, but not all foods are equal.

- The best source of low-calorie carbohydrates are vegetables and fruit.
- Cut-down on bread, rice, pasta.
- Avoid cake, donuts & savouries/pastries.

When we think of carbohydrates, we usually think of bread, pasta, rice and cakes. These are not the best types of food containing carbs because of how they are made. Raw ingredients are so refined during the manufacturing process that the manufacturers often artificially put nutrients back in, along with preservatives and sugar. Ever seen breakfast cereal advertised as containing 'fortified with iron and calcium'. Why do they need to fortify it in the first place? Refined flour used in bread, cakes and pastries is made with pulverized wheat where very little of the natural nutrients survive, but sugar and salt gets added. If you want to eat bread, rice and pasta, try and choose the wholegrain varieties instead, but remember to stay within your calorie limit. Do your best to avoid cake, donuts, pastries and savoury products, as they contain high amounts of salt, sugar and fat. Vegetables and fruits are definitely the best source of low calorie carbohydrates. Don't worry about the natural sugar in fruit. It does NOT count towards the daily limit of sugar we should aim to limit ourselves to.

Protein

Your body uses protein to build and repair skin, muscles, bones and blood. Your body does not store reservoirs of protein, like it does with carbohydrate and fat, so it relies on you eating it. Meat, poultry, fish, eggs and nuts are all good sources of protein and either have zero or very low amounts of carbohydrate.

Fat

Fat has a bad reputation, but it is actually very important for many bodily functions. It is essential for growth and development. It helps absorb and store vitamins A, D, E and K. It protects organs and body tissues by providing cushioning. It supports the immune function and regulates inflammation.

Unsaturated fat is the good type - it can help lower blood cholesterol. This type of fat is found in oily fish like salmon, sardines and mackerel, nuts and seeds, olive oils, and some fruits and vegetables, like avocado.

Saturated and Trans fat are the bad kinds. They can raise cholesterol, which can increase the risk of heart disease. Most people in the UK don't eat a lot of Trans fat in their diet because manufacturers have reduced their use of it. It's the saturated fat we need to be aware of and cut down, found in fatty meat, sausages, pies, butter, hard cheese, cream, ice cream, savoury snacks, chocolate, biscuits, cakes and pastries.

Vitamins & Minerals

Vitamins and minerals are essential nutrients your body needs in small amounts to work properly, which most people get by eating a varied and balanced diet. There are two types of vitamins: **fat-soluble** and **water-soluble.**

Fat-soluble vitamins are found mainly in animal products like milk, dairy food, eggs, and oily fish. Your body is able to store fat-soluble vitamins, like vitamin A, D, E and K, in your liver and fatty tissue for future use, so it's not necessary to eat dairy, eggs and oily fish every day.

- Vitamin A helps your immune system, helps you see in the dark and keeps skin healthy. Good sources are cheese, eggs, oily fish and milk.
- Vitamin D helps control how much calcium and phosphate is in your body, keeping bones and

teeth healthy. Diseases like rickets are caused by a lack of Vitamin D. The best source is sunlight on our skin but it's also found in oily fish and eggs.

- Vitamin E works as an antioxidant, protecting your body, maintaining healthy skin, eyes and strengthens your immune system. Good sources include plant oils, such as soya, corn and olive oil, nuts and seeds, and wheat germ, found in cereals and bread.

- Vitamin K helps blood to clot and there is evidence it helps keep bones healthy. Good sources of vitamin K include green leafy vegetables, like broccoli and spinach, vegetable oils and cereal grain. There are also small amounts in meat and dairy.

Water-soluble vitamins are not stored in the body, so you need to replenish them frequently. They are found in fruit, vegetables, grains and dairy, but unlike fat-soluble vitamins, they can be destroyed by heat when being cooked. The best way to keep as many of the water-soluble vitamins as possible is to steam or grill foods, rather than boil them. Water-soluble vitamins include C, B and folic acid.

- Vitamin C helps keep cells and connective tissue healthy, which supports other tissues and organs. Vitamin C is found in fruit and vegetables, like oranges, peppers, strawberries, blackcurrants, broccoli and potatoes.

- There are different types of vitamin B and they all do important jobs; thiamine (vitamin B1), riboflavin (vitamin B2), niacin (vitamin B3), pantothenic acid, vitamin B6, folic acid and vitamin B12. These vitamins breakdown and release energy from food, keep the nervous system, eyes and skin healthy, allowing the body to use and store energy from protein and carbs in food, help form haemoglobin - the substance that carries oxygen around in the blood and make healthy red blood cells. Good sources include vegetables, meat, fish and dairy. A well balanced diet will provide everything you need.

There are also minerals, like calcium and iron that are just as important. They help to build strong bones and teeth, control body fluids inside and outside cells and turn the food we eat in energy. Minerals are found in meat, cereals (including bread), fish, milk and dairy foods, vegetables, fruit and nuts.

Food Labelling Explained

So, now you know about the different components in the food you eat; carbs, protein, fats, vitamins and minerals. But how do you find out how much is in food and if the levels are unhealthy?

Answering the first part is easy. What's in the food? The food industry is very good are putting the nutritional values on the packaging. Examine the labelling of any food item and look for the number of calories, carbs, protein, total fat, saturated fat, sugar and salt. Looking at the calorie content is essential for this diet plan, since we're trying to stay below a daily calorie limit. Most figures are given per 100g, making it easier to compare different products, allowing us to choose the varieties with the fewest calories. The other things to look for are on the labelling is **saturated fat** (sometimes called saturates), **sugar** and **salt**.

Answering part two, is the food we're eating healthy or not, is not so easy. This is where the food industry has not been forthcoming about their unhealthy products, just the good ones. They don't want their profits harmed if their products are demonised for being unhealthy. So, the food industry leaves it to us to figure it out. The problem is, we don't know how much fat, and sugar and salt is bad for us.

Things are changing and it is the UK supermarkets that are leading the food labelling revolution. They display a traffic light system on the packaging of their own-brand foods, that not only show the nutrient amounts, but they're also colour-coded, to show if the levels are fine, borderline or high. This system makes it much easier to identify products with too much saturated fat, sugar, salt or calories. You don't even need to know the specific values, where these daily limits are, you just interpret the colour-coding. You can easily save calories by comparing products and at the same time, avoid ones with high levels of saturated fat, sugar and salt.

Not all food manufacturers display the traffic light system, so it's good to know some numbers, so you can judge products yourself. This is the information the food manufacturers prefer you didn't know. The three most important numbers to learn are the high levels for saturated fat, sugar and salt that would be displayed as red on packaging.

- High levels of Saturated Fat: **5g**
- High levels of Sugar: **22.5g**
- High levels of Salt: **1.5g**

Comparing Food

In this chapter, I examine around five hundred products and I determine which are good and bad, calorie-wise. I order everything by calories and group them into LOW, OK and HIGH, according to the number of calories they have, per 100g.

Most of the dietary information about food was taken from Sainsbury's website, but I also got information from the websites of McDonalds, KFC, Nando's and myfitnesspal.com.

To make fair comparisons, most food is based on 100g or 100ml. Some of the take-away food at the end is based on portion sizes, which is a very subjective measure, but this isn't a scientific study. You already know that a bag of chips has more calories in it than an apple.

The Good vs. Bad

I group each food by its calorie content, into 'LOW, 'OK' and 'HIGH, based on the following...

LOW

- Any food with less than 150 calories per 100g.
- These foods should be your first choices.

OK

- Any food between 150 - 300 calories per 100g.
- These foods can be eaten, but be sensible about the quantity. We are controlling calories with this diet, so the more 'LOW' foods you can choose the better.

HIGH

- Any food over 300 calories per 100g.
- These foods should be avoided. They just have too many calories.

I also add comments as well, so you can see if any of the food has high levels of fat, sugar and salt. Some products contain a surprising amount of fat, salt or sugar, even if they are packaged and marketed as low-calorie.

I will review...

- CARBOHYDRATES; vegetables, fruit, rice, pasta, bread, cakes
- PROTEIN; fish, poultry, meat (unprocessed), meat (processed), eggs, nuts
- DAIRY; milk, cream, cheese, butter & margarine, mayonnaise, ice cream
- SAUCES & DRESSINGS; chutneys, pickles & relishes, condiments, mustards, salad dressings, tomato, brown, BBQ & other sauces, Worcester & soy sauces
- COOKING SAUCES; Indian, Italian, Mexican, Thai
- TAKE-AWAY FOOD; Fish and chip shop, doner kebabs, KFC, McDonalds, Nando's

Group One
Carbohydrates

Carbs make up some of our most favourite foods. We often eat bread, rice, potatoes or vegetables every day. They fill us up and provide energy, but they come at a cost - calories. Some carbs are more calorific than others.

Vegetables

There are no vegetables assigned to the BAD category, but beware of avocado because it is high in fat (20g per 100g of avocado is fat), which boosts their calorie value. Veggies are the best source of low-calorie carbohydrates. See how few calories there are in the vegetables at the top of this list. Even potatoes are better than rice, pasta and bread.

LOW CALORIE

Celery, 7 kcal per 100g
Cucumber, 11 kcal
Mushrooms, 11 kcal
Iceberg lettuce, 14 kcal
Aubergine, 16 kcal
Peppers, 19 kcal
Tomatoes, 20 kcal
Spinach, 24 kcal
Cabbage, 26 kcal
Green beans, 30 kcal
Onions, 38 kcal
Broccoli, 40 kcal
Carrots, 41 kcal
Garden Peas (Birds Eye), 68 kcal
Potatoes (white), 72 kcal
Sweet corn (Green Giant), 77 kcal
Sweet Potato, 82 kcal
Avocado, 198 kcal

Fruit

All fruits are categorised as LOW, but be careful how much fruit you consume, because they do contain naturally high levels of sugar, which mean calories. Apart from raspberries, all the fruits score AMBER for their sugar level; however, this is not the processed or refined type, so you needn't worry about the natural sugar in fruit being bad for your health. Watermelon and berries are lowest for carbs and calories. Bananas are the worst, three times as much as watermelon.

LOW CALORIE

Watermelon, 31 kcal
Raspberries, 32 kcal
Blackberries, 32 kcal
Strawberries, 33 kcal
Grapefruit, 34 kcal
Pears, 40 kcal
Pineapple, 40 kcal
Plums, 42 kcal
Oranges, 43 kcal
Nectarines, 45 kcal
Blueberries, 45 kcal
Apple (Granny Smith), 47 kcal
Kiwi, 55 kcal
White seedless grapes, 66 kcal
Mango, 66 kcal
Bananas, 103 kcal

Rice

Rice is a lower-calorie choice of carb than bread. Cook-it-yourself rice is better than microwaveable products. Surprisingly, there seems little difference between white and brown rice but the calorie content does vary between brands.

LOW CALORIE

Tilda Brown Basmati Rice, 117 kcal
Sainsbury's Easy Cook White Rice, 117 kcal
Sainsbury's Basmati Rice, 117 kcal
Tilda Basmati Rice, 117 kcal
Sainsbury's Spanish Paella Rice, 118 kcal
Sainsbury's Brown Basmati Rice, 119 kcal
Sainsbury's Brown Rice, 119 kcal
Sainsbury's Thai Fragrant Rice, 120 kcal
Sainsbury's Pilau Rice, 137 kcal
Uncle Ben's Microwave Long Grain, 141 kcal

OK

Uncle Ben's Microwave Rice Golden Veg, 153 kcal
Uncle Ben's Classic Microwave Basmati, 153 kcal
Sainsbury's Long Grain White Rice, 156 kcal
Uncle Ben's Microwave Chinese Style, 166 kcal
Uncle Ben's Microwave Tomato & Basil, 168 kcal
Tilda Steamed Basmati Coconut & Chilli, 181 kcal

HIGH CALORIE

Sainsbury's Arborio Risotto Rice, 344 kcal

Pasta

Whole-wheat spaghetti and lasagne sheets have double the calories and carbs than white varieties. Fat, sugar and salt levels for all these products are fine. Watch portion control though - 100g of cooked pasta isn't a lot. Pasta is not much higher in calories than rice but still better than bread.

LOW CALORIE

Sainsbury's Fresh Egg Spaghetti, 142 kcal
Sainsbury's Whole-wheat Fusilli, 145 kcal
Sainsbury's Whole-wheat Penne, 145 kcal
Sainsbury's Whole-wheat Tagliatelle, 145 kcal
Sainsbury's Fresh Egg Fusilli, 150 kcal

OK

Sainsbury's Farfalle, 160 kcal
Sainsbury's Fusilli, 160 kcal
Sainsbury's Lasagne Sheets, 160 kcal
Sainsbury's Linguine, 160 kcal
Sainsbury's Macaroni, 160 kcal
Sainsbury's Penne, 160 kcal
Sainsbury's Spaghetti, 160 kcal

HIGH CALORIE

Sainsbury's Whole-wheat Spaghetti, 316 kcal
Sainsbury's Whole-wheat Lasagne, 340 kcal

Bread

All the bread I reviewed fell into the OK category. None was GOOD or BAD. However, every single product listed below scored AMBER for salt content. All types of bread are high in carbs and calories. If you want to eat bread, wholemeal has fewer carbs than white-flour varieties, but are fairly similar in calories. The real choice is which type of bread to eat, not whether it's wholemeal or white. Sliced bread is better than muffins, bagels and pitta bread. Wraps have the most calories per 100g!

OK

Sainsbury's Crumpet, 212 kcal
Hovis Wholemeal (medium), 221 kcal
Hovis Soft white (medium), 233 kcal
Hovis Soft white (thick), 233 kcal
Hovis Nimble Wholemeal, 233 kcal
Sainsbury's Muffin, 245 kcal
Weightwatchers Love Fibre wrap, 245 kcal
New York Bakery Plain Bagel, 255 kcal
Pitta (wholemeal), 257 kcal
Pitta (white), 269 kcal
Sainsbury's Wholemeal Tortilla, 269 kcal
Burgen Soya & Linseed, 282 kcal
Sainsbury's Plain Tortilla Wrap, 285 kcal
Mission Deli Plain Wrap, 299 kcal

Cakes

Cake is bad. You can spend your daily calorie allowance on lower calorie food - even bread! They are high in calories, carbs, fat and sugar.

OK

Sainsbury's Strawberry Cheesecake, 260 kcal
Warburton's Teacakes, 262 kcal
Sainsbury's Mandarin Cheesecake, 278 kcal
Sainsbury's Hot Cross Buns, 298 kcal

HIGH CALORIE

Sainsbury's Fresh Cream Donut, 321 kcal
Sainsbury's Cherry Madeira cake, 362 kcal
Sainsbury's Raspberry Cheesecake, 366 kcal
Sainsbury's Muffins, Blueberry, 368 kcal
Sainsbury's Chocolate Cheesecake, 370 kcal
Sainsbury's Madeira cake, 379 kcal
Sainsbury's Angel Cake, 383 kcal
Sainsbury's New York Cheesecake, 393 kcal
Mr Kipling's Jam Tarts, 394 kcal
Sainsbury's Victoria Sponge Cake, 399 kcal
Sainsbury's Muffins, Chocolate Chip, 407 kcal
Sainsbury's Croissant, 420 kcal
Sainsbury's Coffee Cake, 422 kcal

Group Two
Protein

The best sources of protein are animals; fish, poultry, beef, pork, lamb and eggs. If you're a vegetarian, your best sources of protein are vegetables, nuts, eggs and cheese.

Fish

Fresh fish is a great choice. It's low in calories and generally lower per 100g, than poultry and red meat. Fish is also a great source of protein, low in fat and sugar. Most of the products score AMBER for salt. If you want canned fish, only choose the kind in water. Avoid fish stored in oil or tomato.

LOW CALORIE

Sainsbury's King Prawns, 68 kcal
Sainsbury's Smoked Haddock, 98 kcal
Sainsbury's Cod Fillets, 98 kcal
Sainsbury's River Cobbler Fillets, 102 kcal
Sainsbury's Cooked Mussel Meat, 104 kcal
Sainsbury's Tuna in Brine, 113 kcal
Sainsbury's Tuna Steaks in Water, 113 kcal
Sainsbury's Plaice Fillets, 122 kcal
Sainsbury's Scallops, 145 kcal
Sainsbury's Trout Fillets, 149 kcal

OK

Sainsbury's Mackerel in Tomato, 155 kcal
Sainsbury's Sea Bass Fillets, 173 kcal
Sainsbury's Tuna in Sunflower Oil, 189 kcal
Sainsbury's Loch Trout Fillets, 206 kcal
Birds Eye Cod Fish Fingers, 218 kcal
Sainsbury's Salmon Fillet, 229 kcal
Sainsbury's Mackerel Fillets, 239 kcal
Sainsbury's Smoked Kipper Fillets, 255 kcal

Poultry

Poultry is a better choice than red meat. Fewer calories, same level of protein, less fat. Chicken covered in breadcrumbs is high in calories, carbs, fat and sugar. Duck is high in fat which increases the calories.

LOW CALORIE

Turkey: Breast fillets, 127 kcal
Chicken: Breast fillets (corn fed), 137 kcal
Turkey: Steaks, 140 kcal
Chicken: Breast fillets, 141 kcal

OK

Turkey: Meatballs, 164 kcal
Chicken: Drumsticks, 178 kcal
Chicken: Thigh fillets, 188 kcal
Chicken: Breaded fillets, 191 kcal
Chicken: Breaded chicken burger, 192 kcal
Duck: Breast fillets, 199 kcal
Chicken: Hot & Spicy Breaded fillet, 201 kcal
Chicken: Wings, 224 kcal
Duck: Crown, 226 kcal
Chicken: Nuggets, 230 kcal
Chicken: Ham & Cheese Kiev, 230 kcal
Chicken: Southern Fried Mini fillets, 233 kcal
Chicken: Breaded goujons, 244 kcal
Duck: Legs, 246 kcal
Chicken: Garlic Kiev, 281 kcal

Meat (unprocessed)

Choose lean cuts of meat for fewer calories and fat. Beef is generally the leanest, followed by pork. All these products are either AMBER or RED for fat.

OK

Beef: Sainsbury's Fillet steak, 159 kcal
Beef: Sainsbury's 10% fat meatballs, 164 kcal
Beef: Sainsbury's Braising steak, 169 kcal
Pork: Sainsbury's Pork kidney, 173 kcal
Beef: Sainsbury's Lean escalopes, 178 kcal
Beef: Sainsbury's Beef roasting joint, 183 kcal
Pork: Sainsbury's Mince 10% fat, 185 kcal
Beef: Sainsbury's Frying steak, 192 kcal
Beef: Sainsbury's Rump steak, 196 kcal
Beef: Sainsbury's Beef mince 10% fat, 206 kcal
Pork: Sainsbury's Pig's liver, 209 kcal
Beef: Sainsbury's Sirloin steak, 213 kcal
Pork: Sainsbury's Boneless Leg joint, 221 kcal
Lamb: Sainsbury's Diced lamb, 232 kcal
Lamb: Sainsbury's Half Leg, 239 kcal
Beef: Sainsbury's Beef Brisket, 241 kcal
Lamb: Sainsbury's Meatballs, 245 kcal
Lamb: Sainsbury's Half Shoulder, 245 kcal
Lamb: Sainsbury's Lamb's Liver, 258 kcal
Pork: Sainsbury's Pork Shoulder joint, 267 kcal
Lamb: Sainsbury's Mince 20% fat, 269 kcal
Pork: Sainsbury's Pork chops, 279 kcal
Beef: Sainsbury's Rib Eye steak, 296 kcal

Meat (processed)

Avoid sausages, pate, pies, chorizo, salami and pork pies. Choose sliced meat instead. Much less processing.

LOW CALORIE

Salt can be high though. Most scored AMBER for salt, and three of them were RED.

Bernard Matthews Turkey Breast slices, 103 kcal
Sainsbury's Cooked Beef slices, 106 kcal
Sainsbury's Honey Roast Ham, 110 kcal
Sainsbury's Cooked Chicken, Chargrilled, 113 kcal
Sainsbury's Chicken Wafer Thin Sliced, 124 kcal
Sainsbury's Cooked Chicken, Sweet Chilli, 127 kcal
Sainsbury's Cooked Chicken slices, BBQ, 131 kcal
Sainsbury's Cooked Chicken slices, tikka, 137 kcal

OK

Everything in this list is either AMBER or RED for fat and salt.

Sainsbury's Chicken Liver Parfait, 226 kcal
Sainsbury's Corned Beef, 233 kcal
Sainsbury's Chicken Roll, 234 kcal
Sainsbury's Scotch Eggs, 235 kcal
Sainsbury's Duck Liver Pate with Port, 238 kcal
Sainsbury's Chicken & Mushroom Pie, 278 kcal
Sainsbury's Butcher's Pork sausages, 281 kcal
Sainsbury's Chicken & Mushroom Pie, 287 kcal
Sainsbury's Steak & Kidney Pastry Pie, 289 kcal

HIGH CALORIE

The more processing, the worse the numbers get.
Everything is this list is flagged as RED for fat and half
them are either AMBER or RED for salt. All these foods
should be avoided for our diet.

Sainsbury's Pork Cocktail Sausages, 301 kcal
Sainsbury's Ardennes Pate, 301 kcal
Sainsbury's Steak & Ale Pie, 302 kcal
Sainsbury's Brussels Pate, 324 kcal
Sainsbury's Sausage Rolls, 332 kcal
Sainsbury's Spanish Chorizo Slices, 338 kcal
Sainsbury's German Pepper Salami, 340 kcal
Sainsbury's Melton Mowbray Pork Pie, 349 kcal
Sainsbury's Crusty Bake Pork Pie, 350 kcal
Sainsbury's Italian Pepperoni, 368 kcal
Sainsbury's Italian Milano Salami, 398 kcal
Sainsbury's Smoked Chorizo, 475 kcal

If you want a convenient snack, choose slices of turkey,
beef or ham, instead of pork pies, scotch eggs and
sausage rolls.

Eggs

Eggs are low calorie and a good source of protein. With far fewer calories, you can see why eating only the egg white has become popular. Remove the yolk and the amount of calories and fat plummets but carbs and protein remain close to the levels for whole eggs. Poached eggs are quick, easy and don't need oil, like frying does.

LOW CALORIE

Egg whites only, 52 kcal
Mabel Pearman Burford brown eggs, 131 kcal
Clarence Court Old Cotswold Legbar eggs, 131 kcal
Happy Egg Large Free Range, 131 kcal
Sainsbury's Barn eggs, 143 kcal
Sainsbury's Barn eggs, basics, 143 kcal
Sainsbury's Free Range Woodland med, 143 kcal
Sainsbury's Free Range Woodland v large, 143 kcal
Sainsbury's Free Range Large eggs, 143 kcal

Nuts

Nuts are not inherently bad. They contain useful, 'good' fats that are suited to many diets. However, they do possess high levels of calories, so for our diet, it's best to avoid nuts.

HIGH CALORIE

KP Dry Roasted Peanuts, 591 kcal
Sainsbury's Whole Almonds, 595 kcal
Sainsbury's Roasted Salted Pistachios, 602 kcal
Sainsbury's Salted Peanuts, 607 kcal
Sainsbury's Cashew Kernels, 617 kcal
Sainsbury's Salted Cashews, 617 kcal
KP original Salted Peanuts, 619 kcal
Sainsbury's Almonds (blanched), 645 kcal
Sainsbury's Brazil, 699 kcal
Sainsbury's Pine Nuts, 702 kcal
Sainsbury's Shelled Walnuts, 705 kcal
Sainsbury's Pecan, 706 kcal
Sainsbury's Macadamia, 752 kcal

Group Three
Dairy

Milk and dairy products, such as cheese and yoghurt, are great sources of protein and calcium. Choose lower-fat milk, cheese and dairy products to keep the calories down.

Milk

Milk is a good source of calcium, low in carbs, sugars and fat. Skimmed milk is lower in fat and calories than semi-skimmed, which is lower than whole milk. Soy milk and milk made from nuts have the fewest calories.

LOW CALORIE

Alpro Almond milk (Unsweetened), 13 kcal
Alpro Coconut & Rice Milk Alternative, 20 kcal
Alpro Almond Milk (Sweetened), 24 kcal
Alpro Soya light Milk Alternative, 27 kcal
Alpro Hazelnut Milk Alternative, 29 kcal
St Helen's Skimmed Goats milk, 30 kcal
LactoFree Skimmed, 33 kcal
Flora Pro-activ milk, 35 kcal
Cravendale Pure Filter skimmed, 37 kcal
LactoFree Semi skimmed, 40 kcal
Sainsbury's Skimmed milk, 43 kcal
St Helen's Semi skimmed goat's milk, 44 kcal
Sainsbury's Semi skimmed, 46 kcal
Cravendale Pure Filter Semi skimmed, 49 kcal
Lactofree Whole, 57 kcal
St Helen's Whole Goats milk, 61 kcal
Sainsbury's Whole milk, 63 kcal
Cravendale Pure Filter Whole milk, 65 kcal
Sainsbury's Jersey milk, 79 kcal
Graham's Gold Jersey Full Cream, 81 kcal

Cream

Real dairy cream is bad for this diet. It's very high in calories. The best versions to choose are low calorie alternatives, like Elmlea. Crème fraiche and soured cream don't fair too badly.

OK

Elmlea Single Cream alternative, 159 kcal
Sainsbury's half fat Crème Fraiche, 163 kcal
Yeo Valley Organic Half fat Crème Fraiche, 168 kcal
Sainsbury's Single cream, 183 kcal
Sainsbury's soured cream, 187 kcal
Anchor Squirty Cream Light, 195 kcal
Elmlea Light Double Cream alternative, 247 kcal

HIGH CALORIE

Anchor Squirty cream, 345 kcal
Lactofree cream, 350 kcal
Elmlea Double Cream alternative, 351 kcal
Sainsbury's Whipping cream, 367 kcal
Anchor Squirty cream, extra thick, 418 kcal
Sainsbury's Double cream, 439 kcal
Sainsbury's Extra Thick Double cream, 439 kcal

Cheese

Hard cheese is a good source of protein, but it's high in fat, salt and calories. Fine for Atkins, but not good for our calorie restricted diet. Soft, low calorie cheeses like Philadelphia Light have the fewest calories but all three of these products scored AMBER for fat, sugar and salt.

LOW CALORIE

Philadelphia Light Chives, 151 kcal
Philadelphia Light, 152 kcal

OK

Primula Cheese spread, 210 kcal
Sainsbury's Italian Mozzarella, 217 kcal
Philadelphia (Original), 235 kcal
Sainsbury's Greek feta, 276 kcal
Sainsbury's Whole Camembert, 284 kcal

HIGH CALORIE

President Brie, 347 kcal
Sainsbury's Caerphilly, 373 kcal
Sainsbury's Wensleydale, 381 kcal
Sainsbury's Mild Cheddar, 390 kcal
Sainsbury's Red Leicester, 390 kcal
Sainsbury's Mature Cheddar, 390 kcal
Sainsbury's Double Gloucester, 404 kcal
Sainsbury's Blue Stilton, 410 kcal
Cathedral City Mature Cheddar, 416 kcal

Butter & Margarine

Go without butter or use the lowest calorie spread you
can find. High in calories!

OK
Flora Light spread, 281 kcal

HIGH CALORIE
Benecol Light spread, 324 kcal
Bertolli Light spread, 346 kcal
Flora Original spread, 405 kcal
Clover Light spread, 454 kcal
Anchor Light spread, 516 kcal
I Can't Believe It's Not Butter! Original, 528 kcal
Bertolli Original spread, 536 kcal
Benecol butter, 542 kcal
Stork Original spread, 623 kcal
Clover spread, 640 kcal
Sainsbury's Salted butter, 737 kcal
Country Life butter, 737 kcal
Lurpak Salted butter, 739 kcal
Anchor butter, 744 kcal
Country Life Unsalted butter, 746 kcal
Lurpak Unsalted butter, 747 kcal
Sainsbury's unsalted butter, 751 kcal
St Helen's Farm Goats butter, 794 kcal

Mayonnaise

Choose "Lighter than Light" mayo or do without it.
Look at how much the calorie count spikes when you go
from LOW, to OK to HIGH.

LOW CALORIE

Hellman's Lighter than Light mayo, 70 kcal

OK

Hellman's Light mayo, 265 kcal
Hellman's Light squeezy mayo, 270 kcal
Hellman's Chilli squeezy mayo, 275 kcal
Sainsbury's Reduced fat mayo, 279 kcal

HIGH CALORIE French

Sainsbury's French style mayo, 642 kcal
Sainsbury's Garlic mayo, 654 kcal
Hellman's Real squeezy mayo, 668 kcal
Sainsbury's Thick & creamy mayo, 677 kcal
Hellman's Real mayo, 721 kcal

Ice Cream

Ice cream isn't too bad if you're careful. I found two products where calorie levels aren't bad but fat and sugar both score AMBER. 100g is roughly two big scoops.

LOW CALORIE
Carte D'Or vanilla light, 140 kcal
Sainsbury's vanilla soft scoop, 146 kcal

OK
Sainsbury's Neapolitan soft scoop, 164 kcal
Sainsbury's Raspberry ripple, 167 kcal
Sainsbury's Cornish Dairy ice cream, 170 kcal
Sainsbury's Vanilla ice cream, 181 kcal
Sainsbury's Mint Choc Chip, 182 kcal
Carte D'Or Vanilla, 200 kcal
Carte D'Or Strawberry, 200 kcal
Sainsbury's Ice Cream roll, 212 kcal
Green & Black's Organic vanilla, 220 kcal
Viennetta, Strawberry, 240 kcal
Viennetta, Vanilla, 250 kcal
Viennetta, Mint, 250 kcal
Green & Black's Organic Chocolate, 250 kcal
Haagen-Dazs Ice Cream Vanilla, 251 kcal
Ben & Jerry's Choc Fudge Brownie, 260 kcal
Haagen-Dazs Cookies and Cream, 263 kcal
Ben & Jerry's Phish Food, 270 kcal
Ben & Jerry's Cookie Dough, 270 kcal

Group Four
Sauces & Dressings

This is a food group I thought would be bad, but it's not true. There are products in each sub-group that easily fit into the LOW calorie zone.

Watch out for the sugar and salt levels though. Salt in some of the mustards and soy sauces, are the highest I found in all of the tables. Be careful with salad dressings too. The vinaigrettes are a better choice than the creams and sauces.

Chutneys, Pickles & Relishes

Quite a range in calories between these products, so choosing carefully can save you calories in your diet.

LOW CALORIE

All of these score AMBER for sugar and salt.

Geeta's Mango & Chilli chutney, 49 kcal
Geeta's Lime & Chilli chutney, 50 kcal
Geeta's Mango chutney, 51 kcal
Haywards Piccalilli, 51 kcal
Sainsbury's Piccalilli, 76 kcal
Heinz Ploughman pickle, 99 kcal
Sainsbury's Sweet pickle, 104 kcal
Branston Original pickle, 112 kcal

OK

All these products are RED for fat and high in salt.

Branston Small chunk pickle, 159 kcal
Branston Caramelised onion chutney, 169 kcal
Sharwood's Mango chutney green label, 240 kcal
Sainsbury's Mango chutney, 248 kcal

Condiments

LOW CALORIE

These six are OK for calories but Sainsbury's mint sauce and Colman's horseradish sauce score AMBER for sugar and salt. The remaining four all score RED for sugar.

Sainsbury's Mint sauce, 94 kcal
Colman's Horseradish sauce, 108 kcal
Colman's Bramley Apple sauce, 111 kcal
Colman's Cranberry sauce, 117 kcal
Colman's Classic Mint sauce, 131 kcal
Sainsbury's Smooth Apple sauce, 134 kcal

OK

These aren't too bad calorie-wise, considering you're unlikely to use 100g every time, but again fat, sugar and salt is generally AMBER.

Sainsbury's Horseradish sauce, 168 kcal
Sainsbury's Redcurrant jelly, 260 kcal
Colman's Seafood sauce, 294 kcal

HIGH CALORIE

These condiments are high in calories and fat, scoring RED for fat and salt.

Heinz Tartare sauce, 312 kcal
Sainsbury's Hollandaise sauce, 504 kcal

Mustard

LOW CALORIE

French's Classic Yellow mustard, 73 kcal
Sainsbury's Dark French mustard, 120 kcal
Sainsbury's Horseradish mustard, 128 kcal

OK

Warning levels starting to creep up for fat, sugar and salt which all score AMBER.

Sainsbury's Dijon mustard, 168 kcal
Sainsbury's English mustard, 191 kcal
Colman's Original English mustard, 195 kcal

HIGH CALORIE

This one isn't good. RED for fat, AMBER for sugar and salt and high in calories.

Sainsbury's Dill mustard, 440 kcal

Salad Dressings

This is one food category definitely to watch. It's quite easy to cover your healthy salad in a lot of dressing, which can be high in fat, which means calories. Vinaigrette dressings are the definitely the best to choose, but even they score AMBER for sugar and salt. The numbers start going up as the salad dressing gets creamier.

LOW CALORIE

Hellman's Fat free vinaigrette, 48 kcal
Sainsbury's Sweet balsamic dressing, 61 kcal
Hellman's Balsamic vinaigrette, 75 kcal

OK

Hellman's Honey & Mustard dressing, 186 kcal
Hellman's Garlic & Herb dressing, 205 kcal
Heinz Light Salad cream, 236 kcal
Hellman's Thousand Island dressing, 238 kcal
Sainsbury's French dressing, 263 kcal
Hellman's French dressing, 280 kcal

HIGH CALORIE

Hellman's Caesar dressing, 326 kcal
Heinz Salad cream, 336 kcal
Pizza Express Caesar light dressing, 348 kcal
Sainsbury's Caesar dressing, 439 kcal

Tomato, Brown & Other sauces

Choosing carefully which products you buy can save you calories, without having to give them up. Low calorie sugar ketchup is better than regular tomato ketchup, but all are either AMBER or RED for sugar and salt.

LOW CALORIE

Heinz Tomato ketchup 50% less sugar, 64 kcal
Sainsbury's Tomato ketchup, 68 kcal
Daddies Tomato ketchup, 102 kcal
Heinz Tomato ketchup, 103 kcal
Daddies Brown sauce, 108 kcal
Heinz Organic Tomato ketchup, 112 kcal
HP Brown sauce, 122 kcal
Heinz BBQ Classic sauce, 133 kcal
HP Fruity sauce, 135 kcal

OK

Jack Daniel's Original BBQ sauce, 163 kcal
Jack Daniel's Smokey BBQ sauce, 173 kcal
Blue Dragon Sweet Chilli sauce, 184 kcal
Colman's Chunky Burger sauce, 230 kcal

HIGH CALORIE

Heinz Burger sauce, 408 kcal

Worcester & Soy sauces

No need to worry about Worcester and soy sauces. They're low in calories and you'll only use a small amount. Sugar and salt content is AMBER for all but the last two. They score RED for sugar and salt, but you'll never use 100g in one go.

LOW CALORIE

Blue Dragon Light Soy sauce, 51 kcal
Blue Dragon Reduced Salt Soy sauce, 59 kcal
Sainsbury's Light Soy sauce, 69 kcal
Kikkoman Soy sauce, reduced salt, 82 kcal
Blue Dragon Soy sauce, 90 kcal
Lea & Perrins Worcestershire sauce, 96 kcal
Sainsbury's Dark Soy sauce, 117 kcal
Sainsbury's Worcester sauce, 143 kcal

Group Five
Cooking Sauces

Italian, Indian, Mexican and Thai food is very popular and easy to make at home, thanks to the range of ingredients available in supermarkets, but do you know how many calories are in those jars of sauce?

Italian tomato-based sauces are the best because they're full of tomatoes, unsurprisingly. Chilli sauces are next best, followed by curry sauces. Creamy curries, creamy pasta sauces and Thai sauces come out as the worst for calories. So, Spaghetti Bolognese, chilli and meat curries for dinner then!

Italian

Pasta sauces are good, since the biggest ingredient is tomato, which is low calorie. The creamy carbonara and lasagne sauces are all still under 150 kcal per 100g. The best option is to buy the light versions. Every single product scores AMBER for salt content though.

LOW CALORIE

Sainsbury's Tomato & Herb, light, 28 kcal
Dolmio Bolognese sauce low fat, 33 kcal
Sainsbury's Pasta sauce, basics, 34 kcal
Dolmio Tomato & Chilli Meatball sauce, 36 kcal
Dolmio Lasagne Tomato sauce, light, 39 kcal
Sainsbury's Pasta sauce, Onion & Garlic, 41 kcal
Dolmio Original Bolognese sauce, 44 kcal
Dolmio Lasagne Tomato sauce, 47 kcal
Sainsbury's Tomato & Herb pasta sauce, 51 kcal
Loyd Grossman Bolognese sauce, 55 kcal
Dolmio Pasta Bake, Tomato & Cheese, 56 kcal
Dolmio Microwaveable, Creamy Tomato, 57 kcal
Loyd Grossman Lasagne Tomato sauce, 70 kcal
Sainsbury's Pasta bake, Mushroom, 83 kcal
Dolmio Pasta Bake, Creamy Tomato, 89 kcal
Dolmio Carbonara Pasta sauce, 92 kcal
Dolmio Lasagne White sauce, 98 kcal
Dolmio Lasagne Creamy White sauce, 98 kcal
Sainsbury's Lasagne sauce, White, 109 kcal
Loyd Grossman Lasagne Creamy White, 112 kcal
Dolmio Pasta Bake, Carbonara, 123 kcal
Sainsbury's Pasta sauce, Carbonara, 127 kcal
Sainsbury's Lasagne, Cheesy White, 138 kcal

Indian

This was a surprise. Every single product is less than 150 calories per 100g. Every product listed here is AMBER for salt and most are AMBER for fat content.

LOW CALORIE

Sainsbury's Bhuna cooking sauce, 46 kcal
Sainsbury's Balti cooking sauce, 49 kcal
Sainsbury's Jalfrezi, 59 kcal
Sainsbury's Curry sauce, basics, 62 kcal
Sainsbury's Rogan Josh cooking sauce, 70 kcal
Sharwood's Rogan Josh sauce, 75 kcal
Sharwood's Madras sauce, 75 kcal
Sharwood's Bhuna sauce, 76 kcal
Sainsbury's Tikka masala, light, 76 kcal
Sharwood's Jalfrezi sauce, 82 kcal
Sainsbury's Madras sauce, 85 kcal
Uncle Ben's Medium curry sauce, 88 kcal
Sainsbury's Korma sauce, light, 88 kcal
Sainsbury's Biryani cooking sauce, 89 kcal
Loyd Grossman Jalfrezi sauce, 91 kcal
Loyd Grossman Bhuna curry sauce, 98 kcal
Sainsbury's Tikka Masala sauce, 105 kcal
Uncle Ben's Korma sauce, 107 kcal
Loyd Grossman Madras sauce, 114 kcal
Sainsbury's Korma sauce, 123 kcal
Loyd Grossman Rogan Josh sauce, 127 kcal
Loyd Grossman Korma sauce, 128 kcal
Loyd Grossman Tikka Masala sauce, 147 kcal

Mexican

This table is a bit misleading. The packet mixes look bad, but you'd need to use about 3 packets to make 100g, which is unlikely.

LOW CALORIE

The chilli sauces are good - on a par with the Italian pasta sauces. Everything is AMBER for sugar and salt.

Old El Paso Thick 'n' Chunky salsa, 39 kcal
Uncle Ben's Chilli sauce, mild, 54 kcal
Uncle Ben's Chilli sauce, hot, 57 kcal
Homepride Chilli cooking sauce, 58 kcal
Loyd Grossman Classic chilli sauce, 69 kcal
Sainsbury's Chilli cooking sauce, hot, 78 kcal

OK

The packet mixes start to score RED for salt and sugar.

Santa Maria Fajita seasoning mix, 269 kcal
Santa Maria Enchilada seasoning mix, 272 kcal
Old El Paso Fajita spice mix, 289 kcal

Thai

More calories in Thai sauces, than Indian, Italian and Mexican, because they have nuts in the ingredients, to give them the 'Thai' taste. However, they all fall within the GOOD category for being below 150 kcal per 100g. Nearly all of them score AMBER for fat, sugar and salt.

LOW CALORIE

Sainsbury's Thai Red curry, 96 kcal
Blue Dragon Thai Green curry sauce, 100 kcal
Uncle Ben's sweet Thai Chilli sauce, 106 kcal
Loyd Grossman Thai Red curry, 107 kcal
Sainsbury's Thai Green curry, 108 kcal
Loyd Grossman Thai Green curry, 110 kcal
Uncle Ben's Thai Coconut curry, 121 kcal
Blue Dragon Thai Red curry sauce, 121 kcal

Group Six
Fast Food

We know this food group is bad for us, but we still eat it, but how bad is it?

These nutritional values are based on portions, not 100g.

Fish & Chip Shop

There isn't very much which is OK for our diet. One fish cake is OK but who orders one fish cake. Everything else falls into the HIGH group because of their calorie content.

OK

Fish cake, 241 kcal
Small Battered Haddock, 232 kcal

HIGH CALORIE

Saveloy, 330 kcal
Small Cod, 375 kcal
Pukka Chicken & Mushroom pie, 477 kcal
Pukka Steak & Kidney pie, 488 kcal
Battered Sausage, 480 kcal
Pukka Beef & Onion pie, 552 kcal
Chips, 839 kcal

This nutritional information was taken from the myfitnesspal.com website.

Kebabs

Oh no! My favourite and it's really, really bad. No more doner kebabs for me then. These figures don't include the salad topping, sauces or the chips that we have with them.

HIGH CALORIE

Chicken Kebab, 620 kcal
Shish Kebab, 700 kcal
Doner Kebab, 1,006 kcal

This nutritional information was taken from the myfitnesspal.com website.

KFC

Better than fish and chips or kebabs, because we're dealing with chicken, which is a low calorie food. It's the Colonel's secret recipe which includes deep frying, that bumps up the calorie and fat count. Original Recipe chicken falls into the OK band, but don't forget to add up the total calories. Two drumsticks and a thigh are 625 calories. Add some chips and you're approaching 1,000.

LOW CALORIE

Hot Wings, 85 kcal
Corn on the cob, regular, 85 kcal
BBQ Beans, regular, 105 kcal
Coleslaw, regular, 145 kcal

OK

Original Recipe, drumstick, 170 kcal
Original Recipe, keel, 260 kcal
Original Recipe, thigh, 285 kcal
Chicken Popcorn, regular, 285 kcal
Original Recipe, rib, 340 kcal

HIGH CALORIE

Fries, regular, 310 kcal
Fillet burger, 440 kcal
Zinger burger, 450 kcal

This nutritional information was taken from KFC's UK website.

McDonalds

Only three products just make it into the OK band of food, they are the smallest products they make and they all score AMBER for fat and salt. The salad and the hamburger also score AMBER for sugar.

OK

Grilled chicken & bacon salad, 182 kcal
French fries, small, 237 kcal
Hamburger, 250 kcal
McNuggets 6 pieces, 259 kcal

HIGH CALORIE

Cheeseburger, 300 kcal
Chicken Mayo, 319 kcal
Filet-o-Fish, 329 kcal
Fries, Medium, 337 kcal
Bacon & Egg McMuffin, 348 kcal
Chicken Sandwich, 388 kcal
Spicy Veggie wrap, 428 kcal
Sausage & Egg McMuffin, 430 kcal
Double Cheeseburger, 445 kcal
Big Mac, 508 kcal
Quarter Pounder cheese, 518 kcal
Big Tasty, 819 kcal

This nutritional information was taken from McDonalds' UK website.

Nando's

Seeing as Nando's serves chicken, you'd think their food would be good, but it's generally high in calories. Nearly all the products in the HIGH group score RED for fat and salt content. Even red flags for fat on 1/2 chicken, a food that is typically low in fat. I'm guessing it's the marinade sauce that's adding the extra calories.

OK
Mediterranean salad, 266 kcal
Spicy rice, regular, 273 kcal
Caesar salad, 290 kcal

HIGH CALORIE
Coleslaw, regular, 264 kcal
Creamy mash, 270 kcal
Chicken, butterfly, 310 kcal
Chicken, 1/4 breast, 309 kcal
Chicken, 1/4 leg, 314 kcal
Chicken wings x5, 315 kcal
Garlic bread, regular, 336 kcal
Chips, regular, 465 kcal
Butterfly burger, 548 kcal
Chicken, thighs, 561 kcal
Chicken, 1/2, 623 kcal
Wing Roulette, 10 randomly spiced, 630 kcal
Chicken, whole, 1,245 kcal

This nutritional information was taken from Nando's UK website.

Water

After all that bad food, let's end on a good note.

Water is more important than you can imagine. The human body is about 60-70% water by mass!!! It's crucial for the metabolic processes that occur inside you and keeping your organs healthy and functioning. Without water you'd stop living.

- You can go without food for about 3 weeks.
- You can go without water for about 3 days.
- It's that important to our bodies.

Recommendations about how much water to drink vary between 2-3 litres a day. Another measure often quoted is to drink 8 glasses a day, which is about 2 litres. If you drink 2 litres of water every day, you'll be fine.

I have a 1 litre bottle on my desk at work, which I fill up in the morning. Once I've filled it up and drunk it twice through the day, I know I've drunk 2 litres. Not very sophisticated but easy to remember. Don't forget all those cups of tea, coffee, even cans of fizzy drink and juices. They all contain water. Food contains water too.

Are You Hungry or Thirsty?

One very important thing I have learned over the last few years is mistaking thirst for hunger. You know that feeling in your stomach. It's been a while since you ate something, so you go and eat. Soon afterwards, the feeling returns. It's because you're thirsty not hungry. You've just consumed lots of calories, when a glass of water is what your body really wanted. I used to get this all the time because I wasn't drinking frequently during the day.

I've learned when I feel like this, to go and drink a big glass of water. If I still feel hungry after 10 minutes, then my body really is hungry. It's a discipline you'll get into over time.

Feel hungry? Drink water first and wait a few minutes.

Tap Water or Bottled Water?

The nutritional differences in tap water and bottled water are negligible. Bottled water isn't especially healthier for you. The biggest difference is taste. All water contains minerals like calcium and magnesium and dissolved gasses. The differences can be minute, but it's enough to alter the taste.

Tap water is cheap and in the UK, safe to drink. If you don't like the taste, then go for one of the bottled waters from the supermarket. You don't need to go for the expensive brands either. Supermarket own brand bottled water is just as good. Find one you like the taste of.

Chapter Six

Recipes

This is the last chapter to help you lose weight, by suggesting some low calorie meals.

There are lots of books you can buy and information, freely available on the Internet, so I'll just give you a few examples, so you can see low calorie doesn't have to mean soup three times a day.

They will be easy to make too. You won't need to go to Cooking School.

Breakfast

Quick and easy to make breakfast.

Fruit Parfait

Natural yoghurt poured of chopped up fruit pieces.

198 kcal

TOTALS: 36g carbs, 1g fat, 12g protein, 26g sugar

½ large banana, 24 kcal
½ cup of strawberries, 61 kcal
½ cup of pineapple, 43 kcal
½ cup of natural plain yoghurt, 70 kcal

Yoghurt & Granola Parfait

Pour the granola into a bowl, spoon the yoghurt over the top, then add maple syrup on top.

226 kcal

TOTALS: 40g carbs, 6g fat, 6g protein, 21g sugar

¼ cup granola, 113 kcal
½ cup of natural plain yoghurt, 60 kcal
1 tablespoon of maple syrup, 53 kcal

Bacon, Eggs & Mushroom

Poach or boil eggs, don't fry them – fewer calories. Grill the bacon. Fry mushrooms using 1cal cooking spray.

241 kcal

TOTALS: 2g carbs, 15g fat, 24g protein, 1g sugar

2 Medium eggs, 126 kcal
2 Tesco smoked bacon back rashers, 94 kcal
100g Tesco closed cup mushrooms, 16 kcal
5 x Fry Light, 1cal spray, 5 kcal

Shredded Wheat & Semi-Skimmed Milk

An alternative to Shredded Wheat could be 60g of Ready Brek for an increase of 71 kcal.

272 kcal

TOTALS: 45g carbs, 5g fat, 12g protein, 10g sugar

2 Shredded Wheat, 153 kcal
200ml Semi-skimmed milk, 100 kcal
5g Candarel sweetener, 19 kcal

Toast and Jam

336 kcal

TOTALS: 48g carbs, 11g fat, 10g protein, 14g sugar

2 slices Warburtons wholemeal bread, 206 kcal
10g Anchor butter, 72 kcal
25g Sainsbury's strawberry jam, 58 kcal

Lunch

Easy to make homemade food or things you can buy from the High Street.

Homemade Chicken Pitta

Natural yogurt, wholemeal pittas and skinless chicken.

313 kcal

TOTALS: 32g carbs, 8g fat, 26g protein, 6g sugar

1 Tesco wholemeal pitta bread, 160 kcal
1 tsp vegetable oil, 21 kcal
75g Chicken breast (raw), 83 kcal
10g Tomato puree, 10 kcal
10g Tikka Masala curry paste, 30 kcal
15g Low fat natural yoghurt, 9 kcal

Subway Ham/Turkey 6" Sub

319 kcal

TOTALS: 48g carbs, 8g fat, 18g protein, 9g sugar

1 x 6" sub with ham or turkey, 280 kcal
1 portion lettuce, 4 kcal
1 tblsp Light mayo, 35 kcal

Tesco Sushi Variety Pack

345 kcal

TOTALS: 62g carbs, 5g fat, 11g protein, 1g sugar

1 Tesco Sushi variety pack, 345 kcal

Homemade Ham & Egg Roll

348 kcal

TOTALS: 42g carbs, 10g fat, 19g protein, 3g sugar

1 Tesco ciabatta roll, 255 kcal
1 Medium hard -boiled egg, 63 kcal
2 slices x Tesco everyday value ham, 30 kcal

Tesco Prawn Sandwich &

370 kcal

TOTALS: 56g carbs, 5g fat, 22g protein, 8g sugar

1 Tesco Light Choices prawn sandwich, 215 kcal
1 Tesco Hoi sin duck sushi 93g, 155 kcal

Heinz Cream of Chicken Soup & a Roll

434 kcal

TOTALS: 66g carbs, 14g fat, 13g protein, 7g sugar

1 Heinz Cream of Chicken soup 400g, 204 kcal
1 Crusty white roll, 230 kcal

Snacks

Here are some examples of low calorie snacks.

2 Satsumas, 42 kcal
20 Cherries, 80 kcal
30 Grapes, 100 kcal
6 Dried apricots, 100 kcal

Activia Fat Free Peach Yoghurt, 74 kcal
Muller Light Toffee Yoghurt, 99 kcal
1 Weightwatchers chocolate and vanilla mousse, 100 kcal

Packet of Quavers, 88 kcal
Walker's Baked Salt & Vinegar crisps, 100 kcal

1 Fun-size Milky Way, 76 kcals
2 Jaffa cakes, 90 kcal
2 Special K Biscuit Moments: 98 kcal

Dinner

Here is a sample of low calorie dinners that are easy to make and still taste great.

Greek-style Roast Fish (serves 2)

389 kcal per person

TOTALS (per person): 24g carbs, 15g fat, 15g protein, 2g sugar

Heat the oven to 200C/gas 6. Place everything into a roasting tin and mix together to coat everything in the oil. Cook for 15 minutes then turn everything over and cook for another 15 minutes. Add lemon and tomatoes and roast for a final 10 minutes.

400g small potatoes cut into wedges, 328 kcal
1 sliced onion, 20 kcal
2 chopped garlic cloves, 8 kcal
½ tsp dried oregano, 3 kcal
2 tbsp olive oil, 239 kcal
½ lemon cut into wedges, 6 kcal
2 large tomatoes, 64 kcal
2 fresh skinless Pollock fillets (about 200g), 112 kcal

Poached Salmon with Creamy Sauce (serves 4)

336 kcal (per person)

TOTALS (per person): 2g carbs, 23g fat, 23g protein, 0g sugar

Place the salmon in a large frying pan, add ½ the wine and enough water to just cover the salmon. Bring to the boil then reduce to simmer. Turn the salmon over and cook for another 5 minutes, then remove from the heat.

In a second frying pan, heat the oil over a medium-high heat. Add the shallot and stir for 30 seconds. Add the remaining wine and cook for 1 more minute. Stir in the lemon juice and cook for 1 more minute. Remove from the heat, stir in the cream and salt.

To serve, place the salmon on a plate, cover with the sauce and garnish with dill.

500g salmon fillet, skinned and cut into 4 portions, 900 kcal
1 cup dry white wine, 154 kcal
2 tsp extra-virgin olive oil, 240 kcal
1 large shallot, minced, 32 kcal
2 tbsp lemon juice, 8 kcal
1/4 tbsp reduced-fat sour cream, 22 kcal
1/4 tsp salt, 0 kcal
1 tbsp chopped fresh dill, 20 kcal

Prawn, Fennel & Rocket Risotto (serves 4)

384 kcal (per person)

TOTALS (per person): 67g carbs, 14g fat, 26g protein, 6g sugar

Bring the vegetable stock to the boil then set to simmer. In a frying pan, heat the oil, add the onion, garlic and fennel and cook on a low heat for 10 minutes until the vegetables have softened but not changed colour. Add the rice and stir for 2 minutes until the rice grains are hot and making cracking noises. Increase heat to medium and begin adding the stock, a big spoonful at a time, stirring constantly and making sure the stock has been absorbed into the rice, before adding the next spoonful. When the rice is almost cooked, add the prawns and continue adding stock for another 3-4 minutes until the prawns are pink and the rice is cooked. Remove from the heat and stir through the rocket and lemon juice. Leave it to sit for two minutes then serve.

1 vegetable stock cube, 34 kcal
1 litre of water, 0 kcal
1 tbsp olive oil, 119 kcal
1 onion, finely chopped, 39 kcal
1 large garlic clove, finely chopped, 4 kcal
1 small fennel bulb, cored and finely chopped, 27 kcal
300g risotto rice, 1040 kcal
300g peeled king prawns, 255 kcal
1 tbsp lemon juice, 4 kcal
70g bag of rocket, 11 kcal

Chicken Fajitas & Tomato Salsa (serves 4)

442 kcal (per person)

TOTALS (per person): 45g carbs, 13g fat, 19g protein, 8g sugar

Heat the oil in a large frying pan, add the onion and peppers and stir-fry for 3-4 minutes. Add the chicken, paprika, chilli powder, cumin and oregano and cook for 5 minutes or until the chicken is cooked through.

Warm the tortilla wraps in the microwave for 30 seconds.

Spoon one-quarter of the chicken mixture into the centre of each tortilla, add a couple of tablespoons of salsa and some shredded lettuce. Roll up and serve warm.

1 Doritos Mild Salsa Dip 300g, 99 kcal
1 tbsp olive oil, 240 kcal
1 large red onion, thinly sliced, 63 kcal
1 red pepper, cored, deseeded and thinly sliced, 27 kcal
1 yellow pepper, cored, deseeded and thinly sliced, 27 kcal
450g chicken breasts, skinned and cut into thin strips, 499 kcal
Pinch paprika, 5 kcal
Pinch mild chilli powder, 5 kcal
Pinch cumin, 5 kcal
Pinch dried oregano, 5 kcal
4 large wholemeal wraps, 794 kcal
½ iceberg lettuce, finely shredded, 10 kcal

Healthy Egg & Chips (serves 2)

478 kcal per person

TOTALS (per person): 46g carbs, 23g fat, 20g protein, 4g sugar

Heat oven to 200C/ gas 6. Tip the potatoes and shallots into a large, non-stick roasting tin then drizzle everything in oil. Bake for 40-45 minutes or until the potatoes start to go brown. Add the mushrooms then cook for another 10 minutes. Make 4 gaps in the vegetables and crack an egg into each space. Back in the oven for 3-4 minutes or until the eggs are cooked thoroughly.

500g diced potatoes, 410 kcal
100g shallots, diced, 20 kcal
1 tbsp olive oil, 239 kcal
2 tsp of dried oregano, 3 kcal
200g small mushrooms, 32 kcal
4 medium eggs, 252 kcal

Seafood Paella (serves 4)

523 kcal per person

TOTALS (per person): 17g carbs, 12g fat, 42g protein, 8g sugar

Stock: Heat the oil in a large pan on a medium heat, add the onion, tomatoes and garlic, cook for 3-4 minutes then add 2 litres of water and the stock cube.

Bring to the boil then simmer for 30 minutes.

Main: Heat the oil in a large frying pan, brown the monkfish for a few minutes on each side then remove and set to one side.

Add the onion to the pan and fry for 4-5 minutes until it goes soft. Stir in the rice and cook for just 30 seconds. Add the garlic, paprika, cayenne and saffron and cook for another 30 seconds.

Stir in the tomatoes and the stock. Bring to the boil then simmer for 10 minutes. Return the monkfish to the pan and add the prawns, mussels and peas.

Cover the pan with foil and cook for on a low heat for another 10-15 minutes then serve.

For the stock:

1 tbsp olive oil, 120kcal
1 onion, roughly chopped, 39 kcal
½ 400g can of chopped tomatoes, 36 kcal
6 garlic cloves, roughly chopped, 24 kcal
1 Oxo chicken stick cube, 20 kcal

Main Ingredients:

24 peeled King prawns, 136 kcal
2 tbsp olive oil, 239 kcal
500g Monkfish, cut into chunks, 345g
1 large onion, finely chopped, 39 kcal
500g paella rice, 720 kcal
4 garlic cloves, sliced, 16 kcal
2 tsp paprika, 13 kcal
1 tsp cayenne pepper, 6 kcal
Pinch of saffron, 1 kcal
½ 400g can of chopped tomatoes, 36 kcal
270g mussel meat, 225 kcal
100g frozen peas, 77 kcal

About the Author

My name is Martin Harris; I am an IT Infrastructure Project Manager by trade. I'd always wanted to do something more exciting, but computers are all I know. In 2013 for a client, I wrote a big book about setting up IT infrastructure for large sporting events. I really enjoyed the writing process, but I didn't think much more about it until a year later, when we got a dog.

We got a Shih Tzu puppy, which got into all kinds of adventures and scrapes in its first year. A friend of ours casually remarked one day, "Your dog is so funny, you should write a book about all the things she does".

In 2015, I took a break from work and decided to have a go at writing this 'dog' book. I began piecing out the story and started writing. A few months later, I published "Diary of a Little Dog" on Amazon. I'm now writing new material. Some more technical I.T. books but also other titles that will appeal to a wider audience.

If you want to get in touch or learn about my current projects, just visit www.martinharris10.com

Regards, Martin.